Healthy Fitness at Home 2024

Beginner's Routine to Get Healthy

[Pick the date]

Dr. Allison Meadows

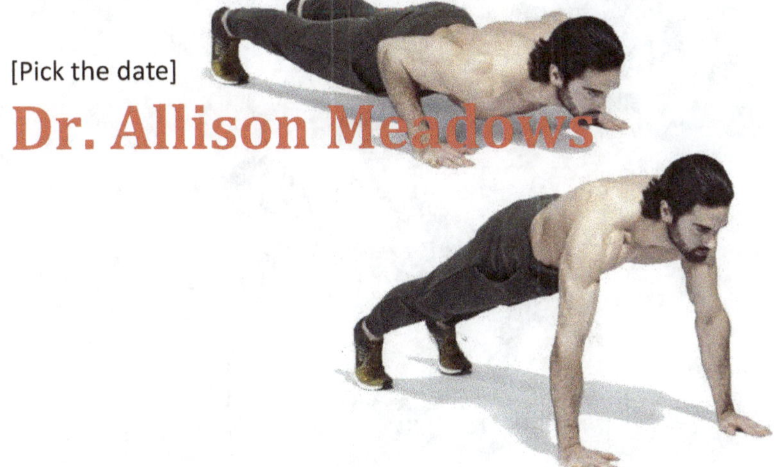

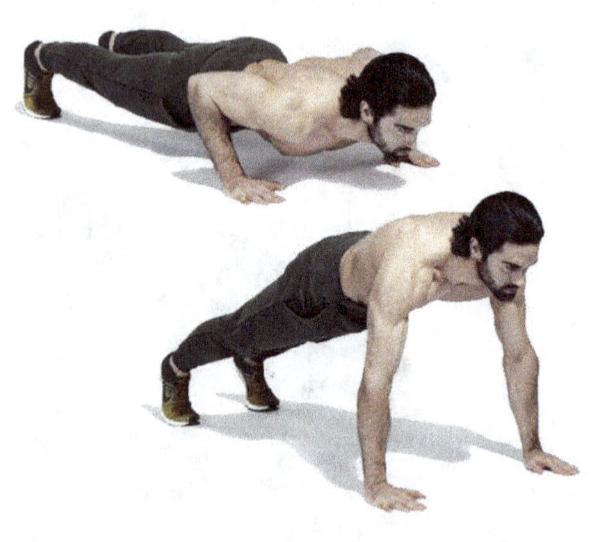

Table Of Content

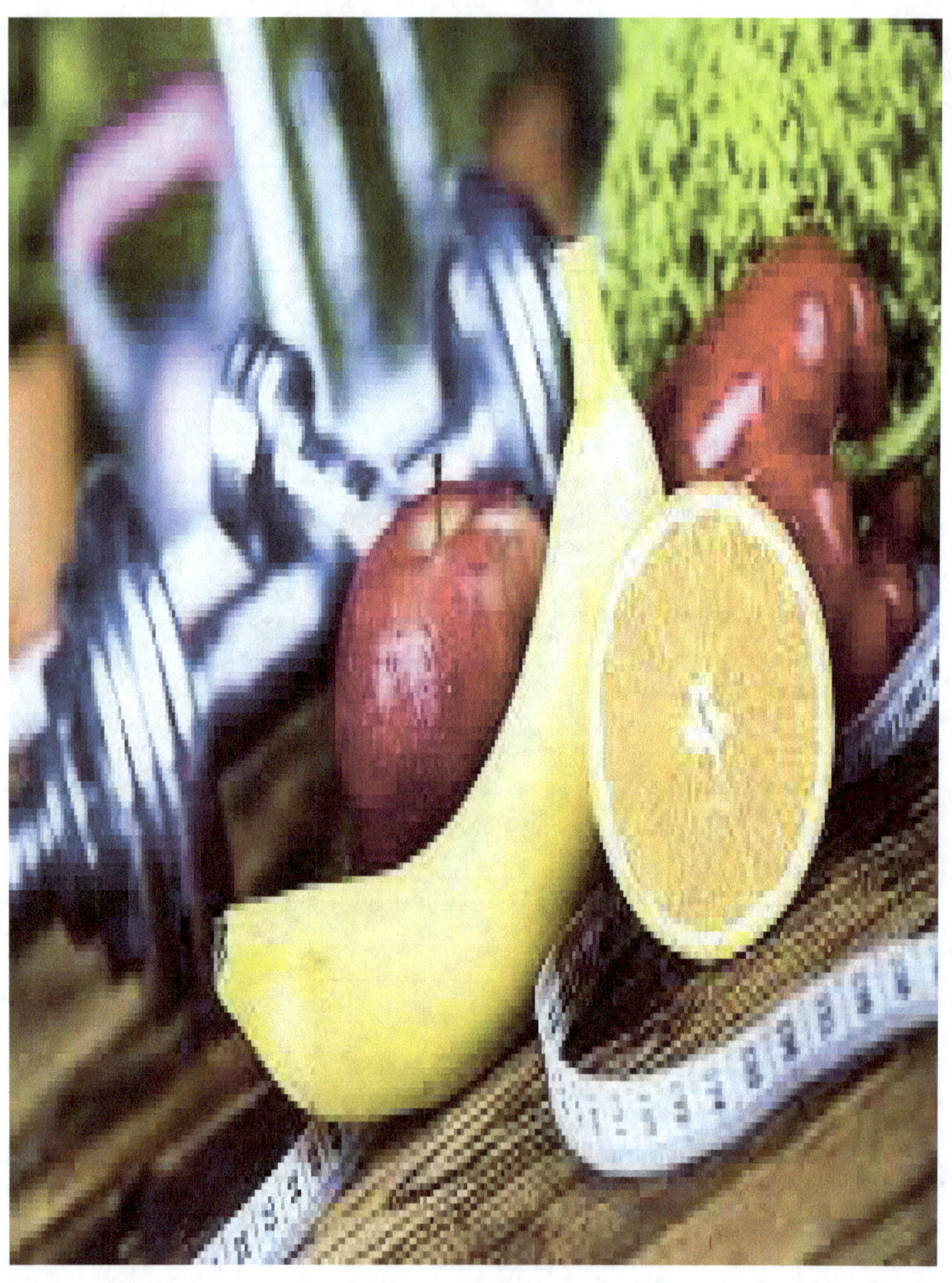

Introduction

Why Fitness Is Essential

Fitness is not just about shaping your body losing weight; it is a comprehensive approach to health and well-being that includes physical, mental, and emotional elements of your life.

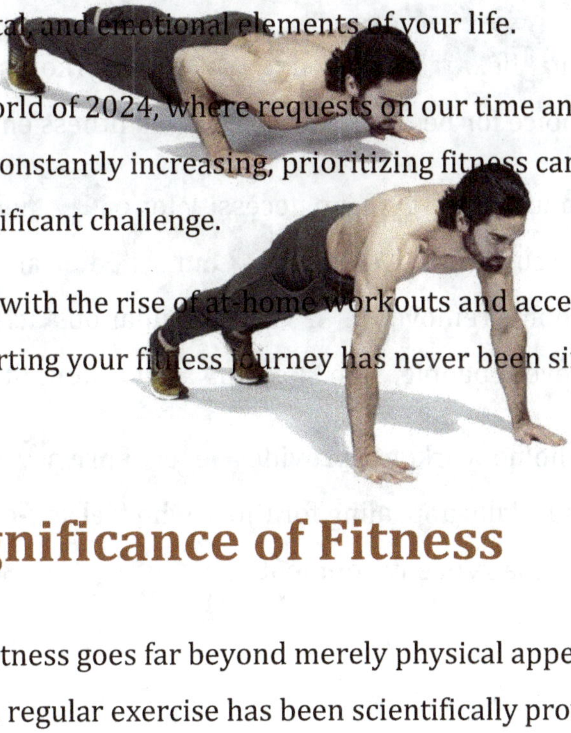

In the busy world of 2024, where requests on our time and attention appear to be constantly increasing, prioritizing fitness can sometimes feel like a significant challenge.

Nevertheless, with the rise of at-home workouts and accessible fitness resources, starting your fitness journey has never been simpler.

The Significance of Fitness

The value of fitness goes far beyond merely physical appearance. Taking part in regular exercise has been scientifically proven to provide a myriad of benefits for both body and mind.

From decreasing the risk of chronic diseases like heart disease, diabetes, and certain cancers to enhancing mood, cognition, and overall quality of life, the positive influence of exercise is undeniable.

In an era where health is a top priority for individuals and societies alike, prioritizing fitness is a proactive move towards longevity and vitality.

Advantages of At-Home Workouts

The comfort and flexibility offered by at-home workouts make them a compelling choice for beginners and seasoned fitness enthusiasts alike.

With no commute to the gym, no necessity for costly memberships and the capacity to customize workouts to your schedule and preferences, exercising at home removes many of the regular obstacles that frequently prevent people from adopting a consistent fitness routine.

Moreover, at-home workouts provide a level of privacy and comfort that can be especially appealing for those who feel self-conscious or intimidated by the gym environment.

Setting Attainable Objectives

Starting a fitness journey without clear goals is similar to embarking on a voyage without a destination.

Whether your objective is to shed weight, build muscles, enhance flexibility, or simply boost your overall well-being, establishing practical and achievable goals is vital for sustaining motivation and monitoring progress.

By setting particular, measurable, attainable, pertinent, and time-bound (SMART) goals, you can construct a roadmap that guides your efforts and holds you responsible along the way.

It is essential to remember that progress in fitness isn't always direct, and setbacks are a natural element of the journey.

By concentrating on the process rather than obsessing solely on results, you'll develop a mindset that is resilient and flexible in the face of challenges.

Filling the Guide with Errors

In the subsequent sections of this manual, we'll delve further into the basics of exercise, explore various workout modalities suitable for beginners, and provide practical tips and strategies for integrating fitness into your day-to-day life.

Whether you're a complete newbie or someone aiming to rekindle their enthusiasm for exercise, this manual will equip you with the knowledge and tools you need to embark on a rewarding and sustainable fitness journey from your own home!

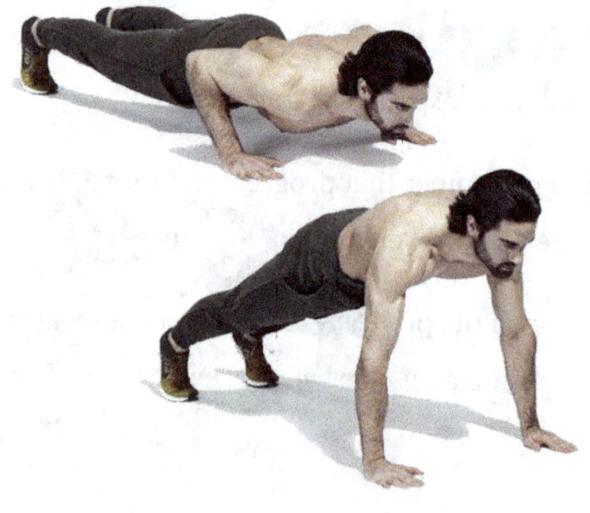

1

Understanding Exercise Basics

Types of Exercises

Exercise can be broadly categorized into three main types:

- ❖ Cardiovascular
- ❖ Strength
- ❖ Flexibility

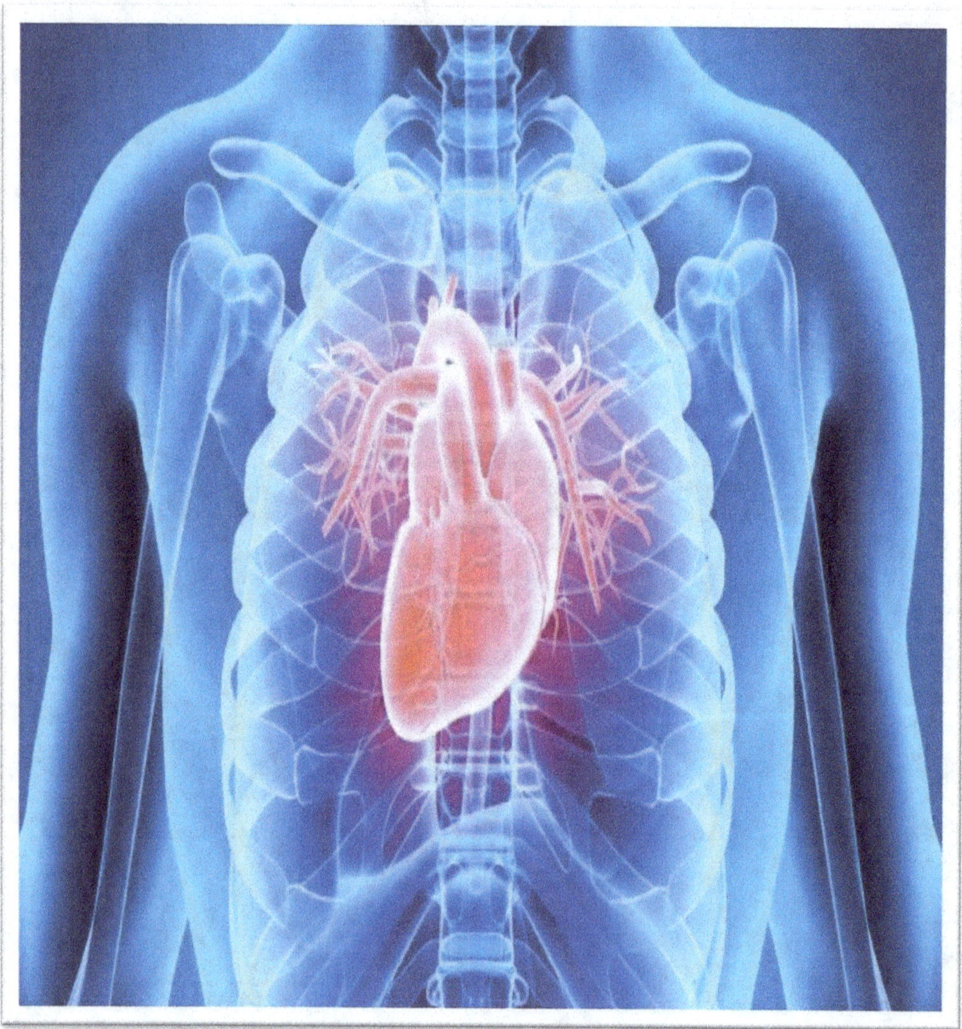

Cardiovascular Exercises

Also known as aerobic exercises, these activities elevate your heart rate and increase your breathing rate, thereby improving the efficiency of your cardiovascular system. Common cardiovascular exercises include:

- ❖ Walking
- ❖ Jogging
- ❖ Cycling
- ❖ Swimming
- ❖ Dancing
- ❖ Jumping rope

These activities not only burn calories and aid in weight management but also promote heart health, endurance, and overall stamina.

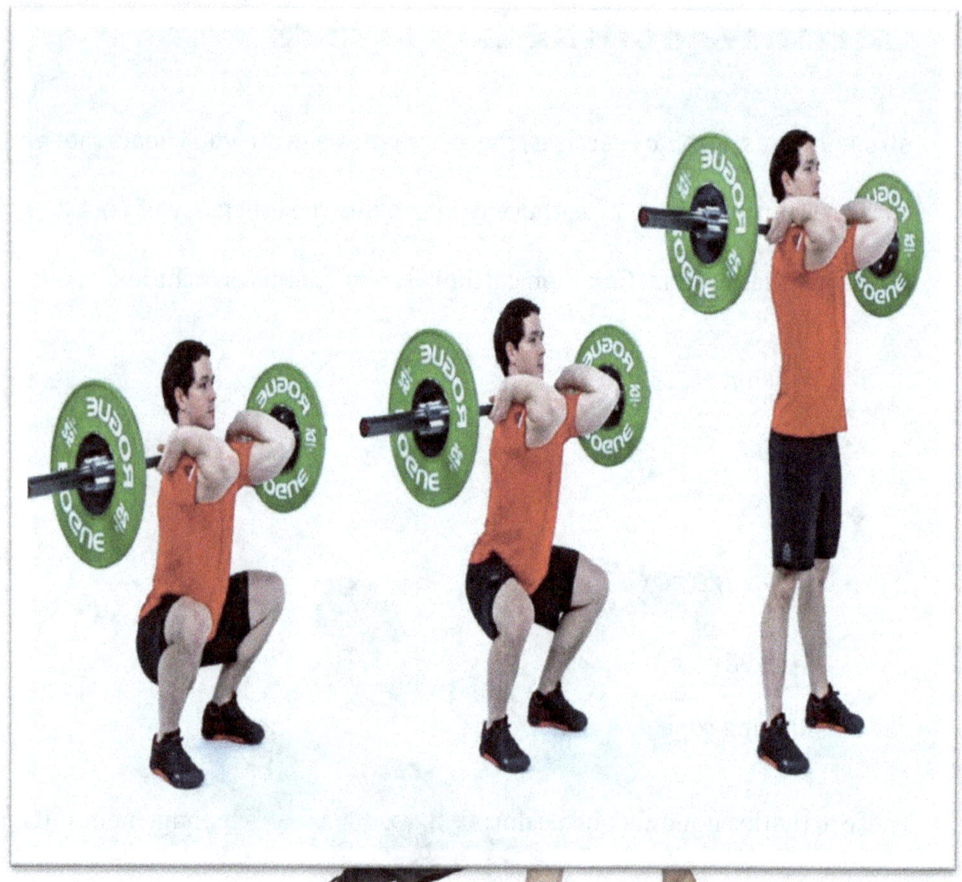

Strength Training Exercises

Strength training, also referred to as resistance training or weight training, involves using resistance to build muscle strength, endurance, and power.

This can be achieved using various equipment such as: dumbbells, resistance bands, or simply your body weight.

Examples of strength training exercises include:

- ❖ Squats
- ❖ Push-ups

- ❖ Lunges
- ❖ Bicep curls
- ❖ Dead-lifts

Strength training into your routine is essential for improving muscle tone, increasing metabolism, and enhancing overall functional fitness.

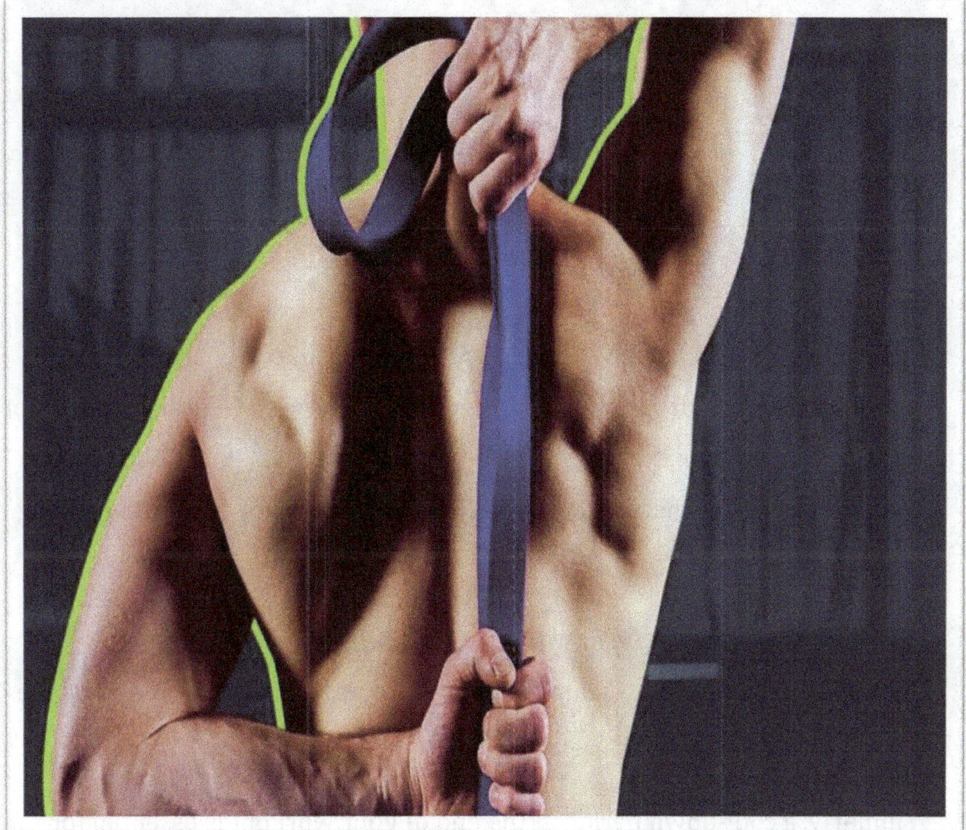

Flexibility and Mobility Work

Flexibility exercises focus on improving the range of motion in your joints and muscles, while mobility exercises aim to enhance movement patterns and reduce stiffness,

- ❖ Stretching
- ❖ Yoga
- ❖ Mobility drills

Are all effective ways to improve flexibility and mobility; these exercises into your routine, you'll reduce the risk of injury, enhance athletic performance, and promote relaxation and stress relief.

Importance of Warm-Up and Cool Down

Before engaging in any physical activity, it's crucial to prepare your body adequately with a proper warm-up routine. A warm-up typically consists of light cardiovascular exercises (e.g., brisk walking or jogging), followed by dynamic stretches that target the muscles and joints you'll be using during your workout.

This helps increase blood flow to the muscles, raises your core body temperature, and primes your body for more intense activity, reducing the risk of injury.

Similarly, a cool-down period at the end of your workout is essential for gradually bringing your heart rate and breathing back to normal, preventing blood pooling in your extremities, and promoting muscle recovery. Cool-down activities may include gentle stretching exercises and deep breathing techniques to aid in relaxation and facilitate the removal of metabolic waste products from your muscles.

Safety Precautions and Injury Prevention

While exercise offers numerous health benefits, it's essential to prioritize safety to prevent injuries and ensure a positive experience. Here are some key safety precautions to keep in mind:

- ❖ **Listen to your body:** Pay attention to any signs of discomfort or pain during exercise and modify or stop activities as needed.
- ❖ **Start gradually:** If you're new to exercise or returning after a long hiatus, ease into your workouts and gradually increase intensity and duration over time.
- ❖ **Use proper form:** Focus on maintaining proper technique and alignment during exercises to minimize the risk of injury and maximize effectiveness.
- ❖ **Stay hydrated:** Drink water before, during, and after your workout to stay hydrated and support optimal performance.
- ❖ **Wear appropriate attire and footwear:** Choose clothing and shoes that provide comfort, support, and adequate ventilation for your workouts.
- ❖ **Seek guidance:** If you're unsure about how to perform certain exercises or have specific health concerns, consider consulting with a fitness professional or healthcare provider for personalized advice and guidance.

Adhering to these exercise basics and prioritizing safety and proper technique, you'll lay a solid foundation for a successful and sustainable fitness journey. In the subsequent sections of this guide, we'll explore specific exercises and workout routines tailored to beginners, empowering you to embark on your fitness journey with confidence and enthusiasm."

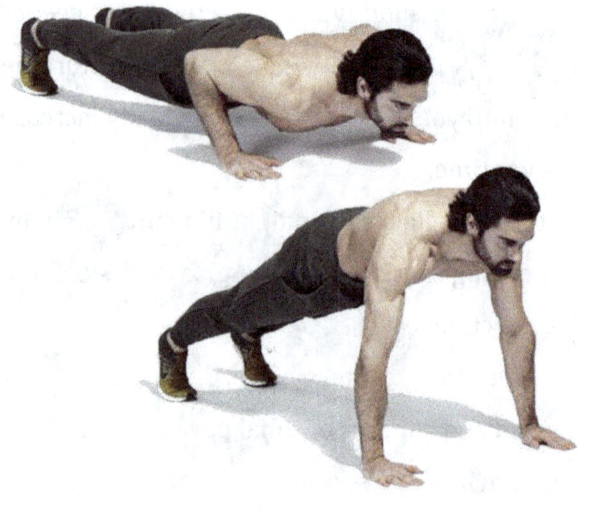

2

Creating Your At-Home Workout Space

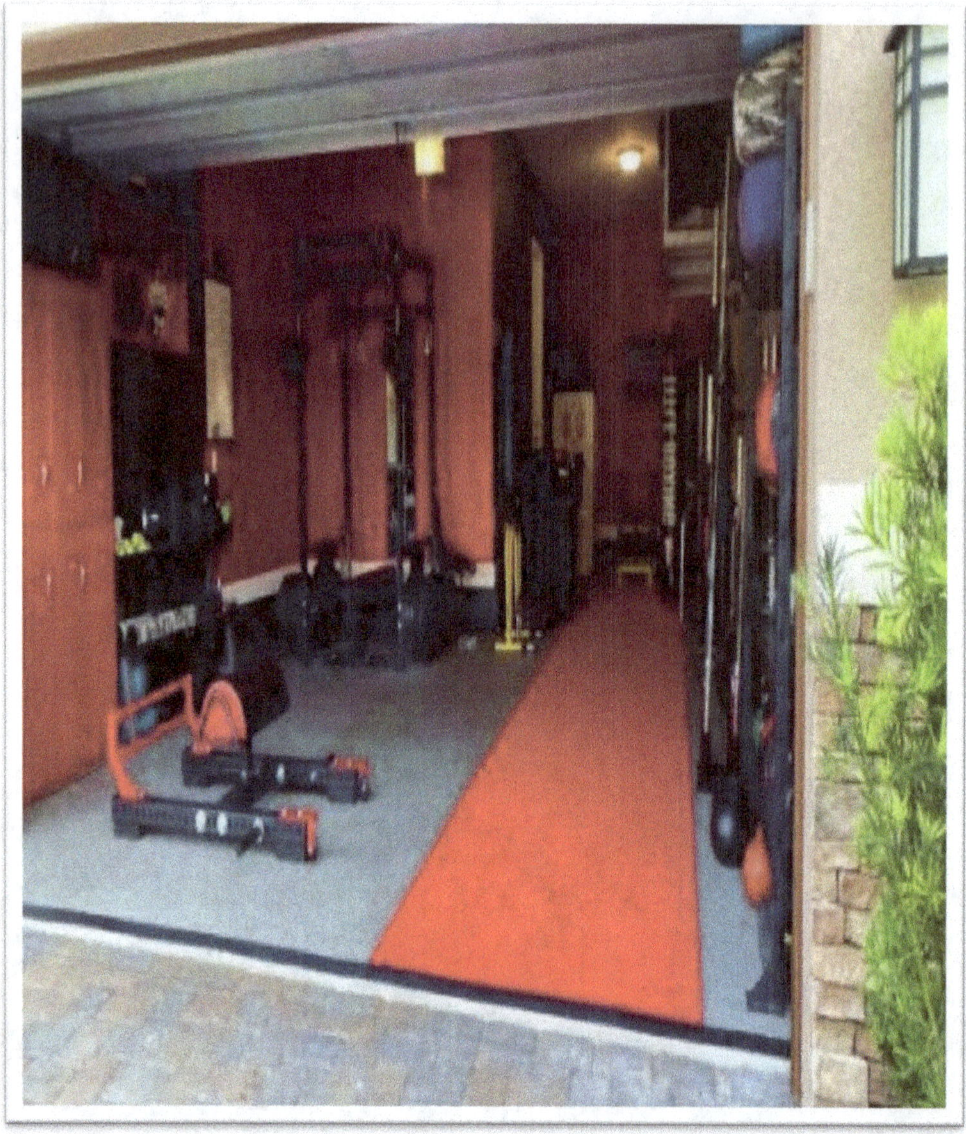

Setting up a dedicated workout space within your home is essential for establishing a conducive environment that promotes consistency and motivation in your fitness routine. Whether you have an entire room to devote to exercise or just a corner of your living room, here are some tips for creating a functional and inspiring at-home workout space.

Choose a Suitable Area

Select a space in your home that is relatively spacious, well-ventilated, and free from clutter.

Consider factors such as natural lighting, privacy, and noise levels to create a comfortable and inviting atmosphere.

If possible, designate a specific area solely for exercise to mentally separate it from other activities and distractions.

Essential Equipment and Alternatives

Determine what types of exercises you enjoy and the equipment you'll need to perform them. This may include items such as:

- ❖ **Yoga mat:** Provides cushioning and grip for floor exercises and stretching.
- ❖ **Dumbbells or kettle-bells:** Versatile tools for strength training exercises.
- ❖ **Resistance bands:** Lightweight and portable alternatives for resistance training.
- ❖ **Stability ball:** Ideal for core exercises and improving balance and stability.

❖ **Jump rope:** Effective for cardiovascular workouts and improving coordination.

If space or budget constraints limit your access to equipment, don't worry! Many effective workouts can be done using just your body weight or household items like chairs, towels, or water bottles as improvised props.

Tips for Making Your Space Motivating and Comfortable

Personalize your workout area with motivational posters, inspirational quotes, or vibrant decor that reflects your fitness goals and personality.

Consider installing a mirror to check your form during exercises and track your progress over time.

Keep your workout space organized and tidy by storing equipment neatly and minimizing clutter.

Create a playlist of energizing music or listen to motivational podcasts to enhance your workout experience and keep you focused and motivated.

Make sure the temperature in your workout space is comfortable and conducive to exercise. You may need to adjust heating or cooling settings accordingly.

Invest in a quality workout mat or flooring if you'll be performing high-impact exercises or activities that require cushioning to protect your joints.

Incorporate Functional Elements

Integrate functional elements into your workout space that facilitate a variety of exercises and movement patterns. This could include:

Wall-mounted hooks or shelves for storing equipment.

An adjustable bench or step platform for added versatility in strength training exercises.

Resistance bands anchored to sturdy fixtures for performing upper and lower body exercises.

A suspension training system (e.g., TRX), which utilizes body weight for resistance and can be easily set up in most spaces

Considerations for Shared Spaces

If you live with family members or roommates, communicate your workout schedule and preferences to minimize disruptions and ensure mutual respect for each other's space.

Be mindful of noise levels, especially if you'll be exercising early in the morning or late at night, and consider using headphones or choosing quieter exercises when necessary.

Thoughtfully designing and organizing your at-home workout space, you'll create an environment that fosters motivation, consistency, and enjoyment in your fitness journey. Whether you're embarking on a solo workout session or engaging in virtual group classes, having a designated space that caters to your needs and preferences will enhance your overall experience and set you up for success in reaching your fitness goals

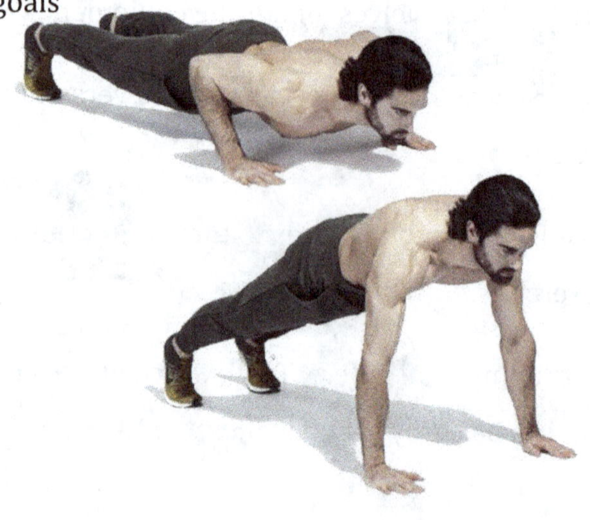

3
Cardiovascular Exercises

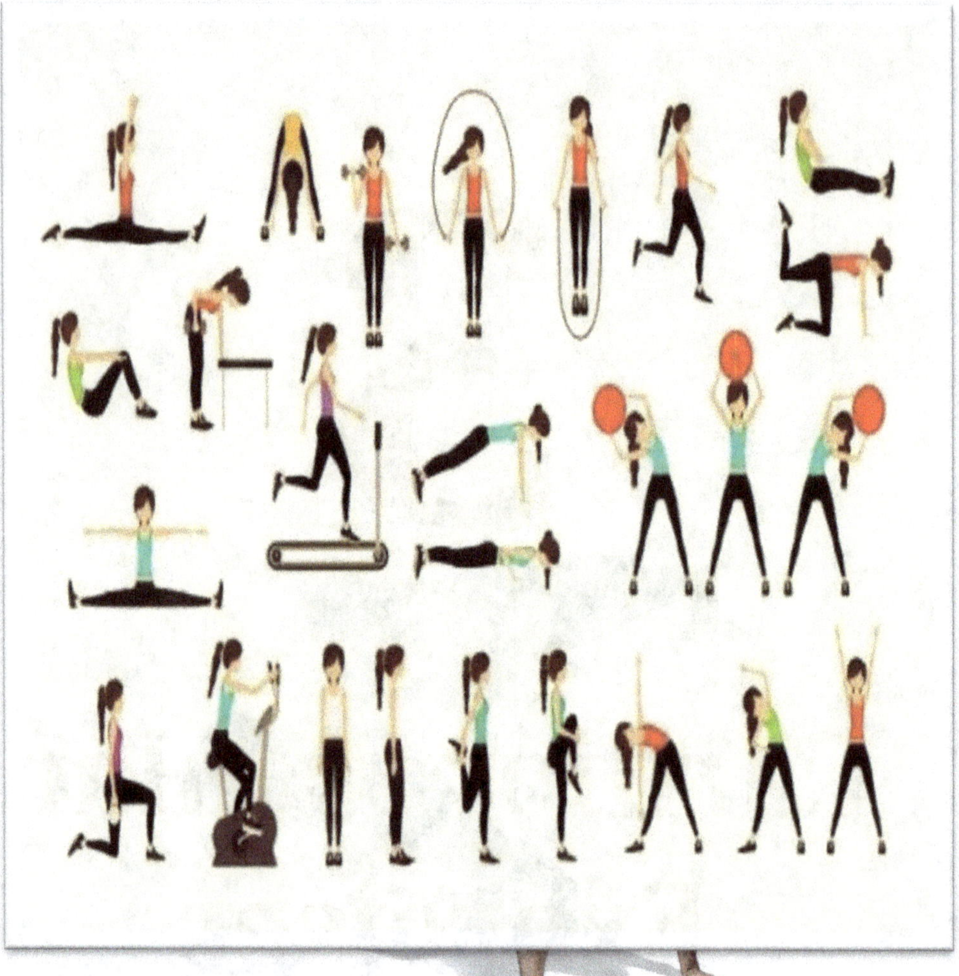

Boost Your Heart Wellbeing and Burn Calories
Cardiovascular works out, too known as cardio or oxygen consuming works out, are crucial components of any wellness regimen. These exercises lift your heart rate, increment your breathing rate, and work expansive muscle bunches, coming about in various wellbeing benefits, counting progressed cardiovascular wellbeing, expanded continuance, upgraded calorie burn, and decreased stretch levels. Whether you're pointing to lose weight, move forward your generally wellness, or basically boost your temperament,

consolidating cardiovascular works out into your schedule is key to accomplishing your objectives. Here's a comprehensive outline of a few successful cardiovascular works out you can do at home.

- ❖ **Jumping Rope:** Jumping rope is a straightforward however profoundly compelling cardiovascular workout that requires negligible gear and space. It's a fabulous way to raise your heart rate, progress coordination, and improve dexterity. Begin with brief interims of bouncing rope, slowly expanding the term as your wellness level makes strides. Varieties such as twofold under or rotating foot designs can include assortment and challenge to your workout.

- ❖ **High Knees:** High knees are an energetic, full-body work out that locks in the center, legs, and cardiovascular framework. Stand input and lift your knees towards your chest on the other hand, keeping up a brisk pace. Center on driving your arms in match up with your legs to maximize calorie burn and raise your heart rate. This work out can be performed for time or as portion of a circuit preparing routine.

- ❖ **Jogging in Place:** Jogging is a helpful and open way to get your heart pumping and burn calories without the requiring any hardware or a huge space. Essentially lift your knees and run on the spot, guaranteeing a light, bouncy movement to lock in your lower body muscles and raise your heart rate. You can shift the concentrated by expanding the speed or consolidating developments such as tall knees or butt kicks.

❖ **Dancing:** Dancing is not as it were a fun and pleasant way to get your heart rate up but too a compelling shape of cardiovascular workout.

Whether you favor hip-hop, salsa, or Zumba, moving permits you to express yourself whereas procuring the benefits of oxygen consuming action.

Take after along with online move instructional exercises or wrench up your favorite music and let free in the consolation of your claim home.

❖ **Stair Climbing:** If you have stairs in your domestic, stair climbing is an amazing way to challenge your cardiovascular framework and fortify your lower body muscles. Basically walk or run up and down the stairs more than once, centering on keeping up great pose and utilizing your arms to help with force. For an included challenge, attempt taking the stairs two at a time or consolidating interims of stair sprints.

❖ **Interval Training:** Interval preparing includes rotating between periods of high-intensity work out and dynamic recuperation or rest.

This approach not as it were maximizes calorie burn amid the workout but too boosts digestion system and progresses cardiovascular wellness. You can consolidate interims into any cardio work out, such as sprinting for 30 seconds taken after by strolling or running for 60 seconds, and rehash for numerous rounds.

Incorporate an assortment of cardiovascular works out into your at-home workout schedule to keep things curiously and challenge your body in diverse ways. Point for at slightest 150 minutes of moderate-intensity cardio work out per week, or 75 minutes of vigorous-intensity work out, as prescribed by wellbeing specialists.

With consistency and devotion, you'll before long encounter the various benefits of cardiovascular workout, from expanded vitality and stamina, to made strides heart wellbeing and generally well-being.

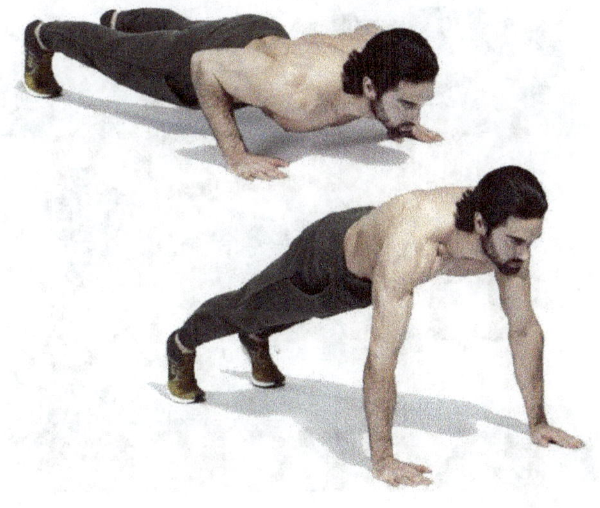

4

Strength Training Exercises

Build Muscle and Boost Strength at Ho

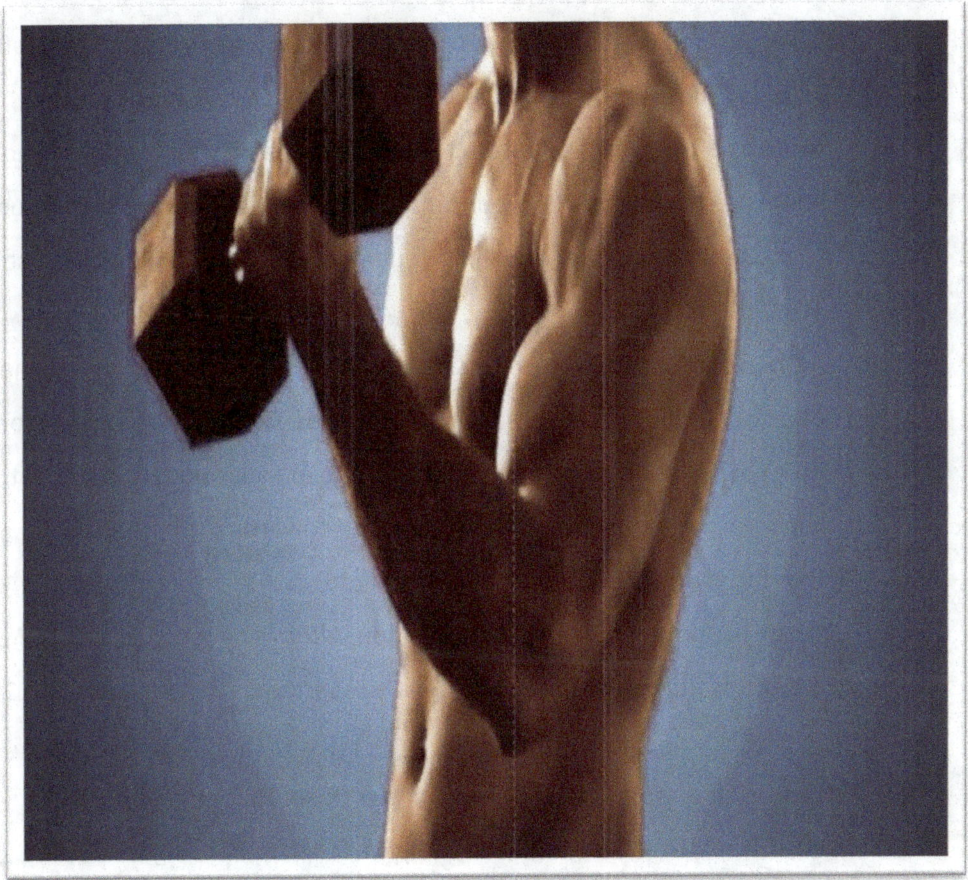

Quality preparing, too known as resistance preparing or toning, is a vital element of any heartiness authority. By challenging your muscles against resistance, quality preparing not as it were builds muscle mass and supplements quality but too upgrades bone consistence, digestion system, and generally utilitarian heartiness. Whether you are an apprentice or a set spa-goer, joining quality preparing works out into your at- home drill schedule can offer backing you negotiate your heartiness objects and move forward your physical prosecution. There are many feasible qualities preparing workshop that you can do at home.

- ❖ **Bodyweight Squats:** Bodyweight syllables are an essential lower body work out that targets the quadriceps, hamstrings, glutes, and pins. Stand with your bases shoulder- range separated, lower your hips back and down as if sitting into a fantastic president, keeping your casket up and your knees following over your toes. Thrust through your heels to return to the morning position, crushing your glutes at the beat. Point for 3 sets 10- 15 reiterations.
- ❖ **Push- Ups:** Push- ups are a classic upper body work out that targets the casket, shoulders, triceps, and center muscles. Begin in a board position with your hands shoulder- range separated and your body in a straight line from head to heels. Lower your casket towards the bottom by twisting your elbows, keeping them near to your body, at that point thrust back over to the morning position. Alter as needed by performing drive- ups from your knees or against a separator. Point for 3 sets 8- 12 reiterations.
- ❖ **Lunges:** jabs are a flexible lower body work out that targets the quadriceps, hamstrings, glutes, and pins. Start by standing with your bases hip- range separated, step forward with one bottom and lower your body until both knees are bowed at a 90- degree point, guaranteeing your front knee remains acclimated with your lower leg. Thrust through your frontal heel to return to the morning position, at that point reappraisal on the other side. Point for 3 sets 10- 12 redundancy per leg.
- ❖ **Planks:** Planks are a profoundly feasible core- strengthening work out that also cinch in the shoulders, casket, and back muscles. Begin in a

drive-up position with your hands specifically beneath your shoulders and your body in a straight line from head to heels. Cinch in your center muscles and hold this position for as long as conceivable, pointing for at fewest 30- 60 seconds. To make it less demanding, you can perform boards from your lower arms or perhaps than your hands.

- ❖ **Dumbbell Exercises:** still, you can perform a multifariousness of quality preparing works out to target distinctive muscle bunches, if you have get to dumbbells or other weighted objects at domestic. Illustrations include:
    - ❖ Dumbbell Lines Targets the reverse, shoulders, and biceps.
    - ❖ Dumbbell casket Press Targets the casket, shoulders, and triceps.
    - ❖ Dumbbell Bear Press Targets the shoulders and triceps.
    - ❖ Dumbbell Bicep Twists Targets the biceps.
    - ❖ Dumbbell Triceps Expansions Targets the triceps.

Choose a weight that permits you to perform 8- 12 redundancies with great frame for each work out, and point for 2- 3 sets per exercise.

- ❖ **Resistance Band Exercises:** Resistance groups are flexible and accessible instruments that can be employed to include resistance to bodyweight works out or image the resistance given by conventional toning gear. Cases of resistance band works out include:
    - ❖ Band Pull- Apart Targets the shoulders and upper back.
    - ❖ Band casket Press Targets the casket and triceps.
    - ❖ Band Columns Targets the reverse and biceps.

❖ Band Squats Targets the lower body muscles.

Acclimatize the pressure of the resistance band to coordinate your quality position, and point for 2- 3 sets of 10- 15 repetitions for each exercise.

Incorporate a combination of these quality preparing works out into your at- home drill schedule, pointing to work all major muscle bunches at fewest 2- 3 times per week.

Keep in mind to begin with lighter weights or resistance situations if you are ultramodern to quality preparing, and sluggishly proliferation the escalated as you gotten to be more predicated and more comfortable with the workshop out.

With thickness and devotion, you will construct muscle, proliferation quality, and move forward your generally physical heartiness from the consolation of your claim domestic.

5

Flexibility and Mobility Work

Enhancing Movement and Preventing Injury

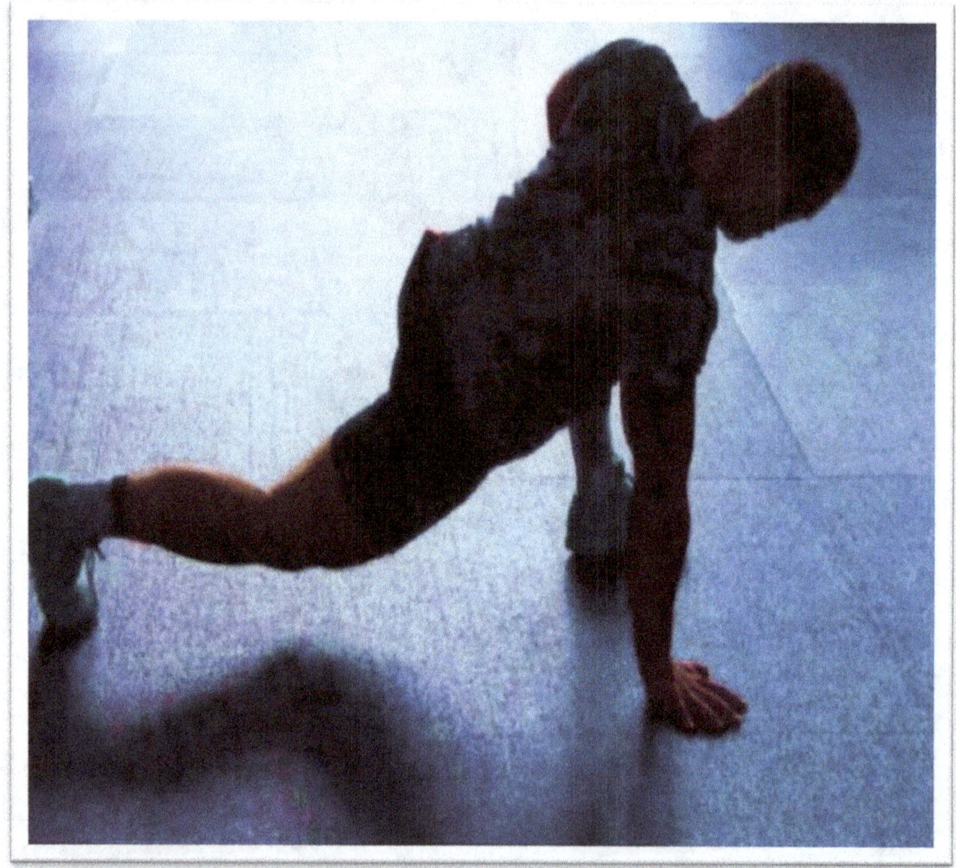

Flexibility and mobility are crucial components of physical fitness that often go overlooked. While flexibility refers to the ability of your muscles to stretch and lengthen, mobility encompasses the range of motion in your joints and the ability to move freely and efficiently.

Flexibility and mobility exercises into your workout routine can improve posture, reduce the risk of injury, enhance athletic performance, and promote overall well-being. Here's a comprehensive guide to incorporating flexibility and mobility work into your at-home workouts.

Stretching Routine (Full Body)

A comprehensive stretching routine targets major muscle groups throughout your body, promoting flexibility and relieving muscle tension. Focus on dynamic stretches before your workout to warm up your muscles and prepare them for movement, and static stretches afterward to increase flexibility and aid in muscle recovery.

Key stretches to include in your routine may target the hamstrings, quadriceps, calves, hips, chest, shoulders, and back. Hold each stretch for 15-30 seconds, breathing deeply and gradually increasing the stretch as tolerated.

Yoga Poses for Beginners

Yoga is a powerful practice that combines movement, breath, and mindfulness to improve flexibility, strength, and balance. Incorporating beginner-friendly yoga poses into your routine can help increase mobility in your joints, enhance relaxation, and reduce stress levels.

Start with basic poses such as downward-facing dog, child's pose, cat-cow stretch, seated forward fold, and warrior poses. Focus on proper alignment and listen to your body, modifying poses as needed to suit your comfort level and ability.

Foam Rolling Techniques

Foam rolling, also known as self-myofascial release, is a form of self-massage that targets tight muscles and connective tissue (fascia) to improve mobility and reduce muscle soreness. Using a foam roller or massage ball, apply gentle pressure to specific areas of your body, rolling back and forth to release tension and increase blood flow.

Focus on areas of tightness or discomfort, such as the calves, hamstrings, quadriceps, IT band, glutes, and upper back. Incorporate foam rolling into your post-workout routine or as needed throughout the day to alleviate muscle tightness and improve flexibility.

Mobility Drills

Mobility drills involve dynamic movements that focus on improving joint mobility and range of motion. These exercises help lubricate the joints, activate stabilizing muscles, and improve movement patterns, making them essential for injury prevention and functional fitness.

Mobility drills such as hip circles, shoulder circles, leg swings, arm swings, spinal rotations, and wrist circles into your warm-up or as standalone exercises throughout your workout. Perform each drill smoothly and deliberately, moving through the full range of motion without forcing or straining.

Breath-work and Mindfulness

Mindful breathing techniques can enhance the effectiveness of flexibility and mobility exercises by promoting relaxation, reducing tension, and improving body awareness. Incorporate deep breathing exercises, such as diaphragmatic breathing or box breathing, into your stretching or yoga practice to calm the nervous system and deepen your connection to your body.

Focus on breathing deeply and evenly, allowing each inhale and exhale to guide your movements and release tension from tight muscles.

By integrating flexibility and mobility work into your at-home workout routine, you'll not only improve your physical performance but also cultivate a deeper sense of body awareness and well-being.

Consistency is key, so aim to incorporate these exercises into your daily or weekly routine to reap the full benefits over time. Listen to your body, be patient with your progress, and enjoy the journey of discovering greater freedom and ease of movement in your body.

6

Sample Workouts for At-Home Fitness

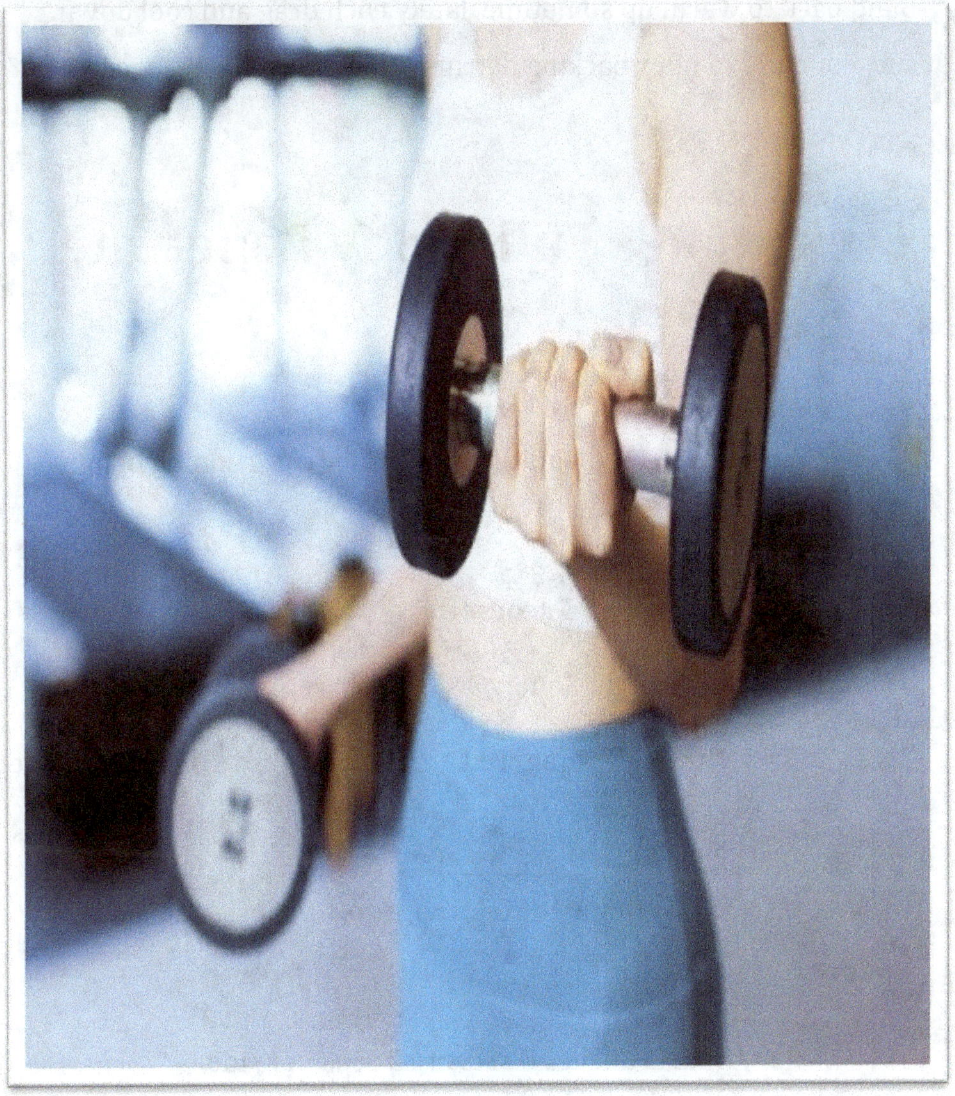

Making a systematized drag arrange is abecedarian for remaining agreeable and negotiating your heartiness demands. Under are test access schedules outlined for apprentices to halfway individualities looking to get fit at domestic? These schedules consolidate a mix of cardiovascular workshop out, quality preparing, harshness work, and portability drills to allow a well- acclimated heartiness hassle.

Band back to warm up sometime, lately each drag and cool down subsequently to offer backing detriment and advance recovery.

Freshman's Full- Body Penetrate Routine

- ❖ **Warm-Up:** 5- 10 beats of light cardio (e.g., running in put, bouncing jacks)
    - ❖ Energetic stretches (e.g., arm circles, leg swings)
- ❖ **Drill:** Bodyweight Squats 3 sets of 12 reps
    - ❖ Thrust- Ups (altered or conventional) 3 sets of 8- 12 reps
    - ❖ Traces (scattering legs) 3 sets of 12 reps per leg
    - ❖ Board Hold for 30 seconds to 1 nanosecond
    - ❖ Hopping Jacks 3 sets of 30 seconds
    - ❖ Bike Crunches 3 sets of 12 reps per side
- ❖ **Cool Down:** 5- 10 beats of light cardio (e.g., walking) stationary extends fastening on major muscle groups (e.g., hamstring extend, casket stretch)

Cardio Circuit Workout

- ❖ **Warm-Up:** 5- 10 beats of brisk tromping or jogging Dynamic stretches (e.g., leg swings, arm circles)

- ❖ **Circuit:** Hop Rope 1 nanosecond

  - ❖ Altitudinous Knees 30 seconds

  - ❖ Mountain rovers 30 seconds

  - ❖ Burpees 1 nanosecond

  - ❖ Bouncing Jacks 1 nanosecond

  - ❖ Rest 1- 2 beats (duplication circuit 2- 3 times)

- ❖ **Cool Down:** 5- 10 beats of tromping or delicate jogging

  - ❖ Stationary extends bending on lower body and center muscles

Upper Body Quality Routine

- ❖ **Warm-Up:** 5- 10 beats of light cardio (e.g., walking in put, arm circles)

- ❖ Dynamic extends fastening on the shoulders, arms, and upper back

- ❖ **Drill:** Thrust- Ups (altered or conventional) 3 sets of 8- 12 reps

  - ❖ Dumbbell Bicep twists 3 sets of 10- 12 reps

  - ❖ Dumbbell Bear Press 3 sets of 10- 12 reps

  - ❖ Bowed- Over Lines (with dumbbells or resistance groups) 3 sets of 10- 12 reps

  - ❖ Triceps Plunges (exercising a strong president or seat) 3 sets of 8- 12 reps

- ❖ **Cool Down:** 5- 10 beats of light cardio (e.g., walking)

  - ❖ Stationary extends fastening on the casket, shoulders, arms, and upper back

Lower Body Quality Routine

- ❖ **Warm-Up:** 5- 10 beats of light cardio (e.g., walking in put, leg swings)

  - ❖ Energetic extends securing on the hips, knives, and legs

- ❖ **Drill:** Bodyweight Squats 3 sets of 12 reps

  - ❖ spots (mixing legs) 3 sets of 12 reps per leg

  - ❖ Dumbbell Romanian Deadlifts 3 sets of 10- 12 reps

  - ❖ Shin Raises 3 sets of 15- 20 reps

  - ❖ Glutes islands 3 sets of 12 reps

- ❖ **Cool Down:** 5- 10 beats of tromping or tender jogging

  - • Stationary extends fastening on the quadriceps, hamstrings, legs, and glutes

Core buttressing Routine

- ❖ **Warm-Up:** 5- 10 beats of light cardio (e.g., walking in put, middle twists)

  - ❖ Energetic extends securing on the center muscles

- ❖ **Drill:** Board Hold for 30 seconds to 1 nanosecond

  - ❖ Russian Turns (with or without weight) 3 sets of 12 reps per side

  - ❖ Bike Crunches 3 sets of 12 reps per side

  - ❖ Leg Raises 3 sets of 10- 12 reps

  - ❖ Superman Hold for 30 seconds to 1 nanosecond

- ❖ **Cool Down:** 5- 10 beats of tromping or tender jogging

  - ❖ Stationary extends fastening on the center muscles (e.g., cat- bovine extend, child's disguise)

❖ **Notes:** Perform each work out with licit shape and design to offer backing detriment and maximize effectiveness.

  ❖ Begin with lighter weights or kinds as requested, sluggishly including escalated and resistance as you comes more predicated and more comfortable with the exercises.

  ❖ Rest for 30- 60 seconds between sets and 1- 2 beats between workshop out to permit for respectable recovery.

  ❖ Hear to your body and alter works out or dwindle escalated as requested to suit your heartiness position and any being injuries or limitations.

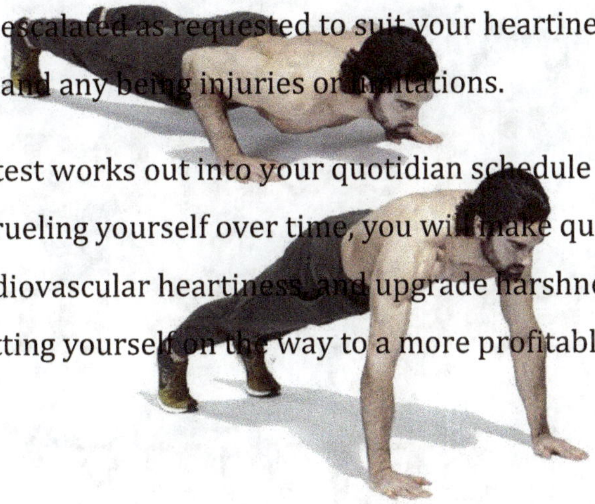

Joining these test works out into your quotidian schedule and impulsively grueling yourself over time, you will make quality, meliorate cardiovascular heartiness, and upgrade harshness and versatility, setting yourself on the way to a more profitable and more dynamic life

7

Tracking Progress and Staying Motivated

Keys to Sustaining Your Fitness Journey

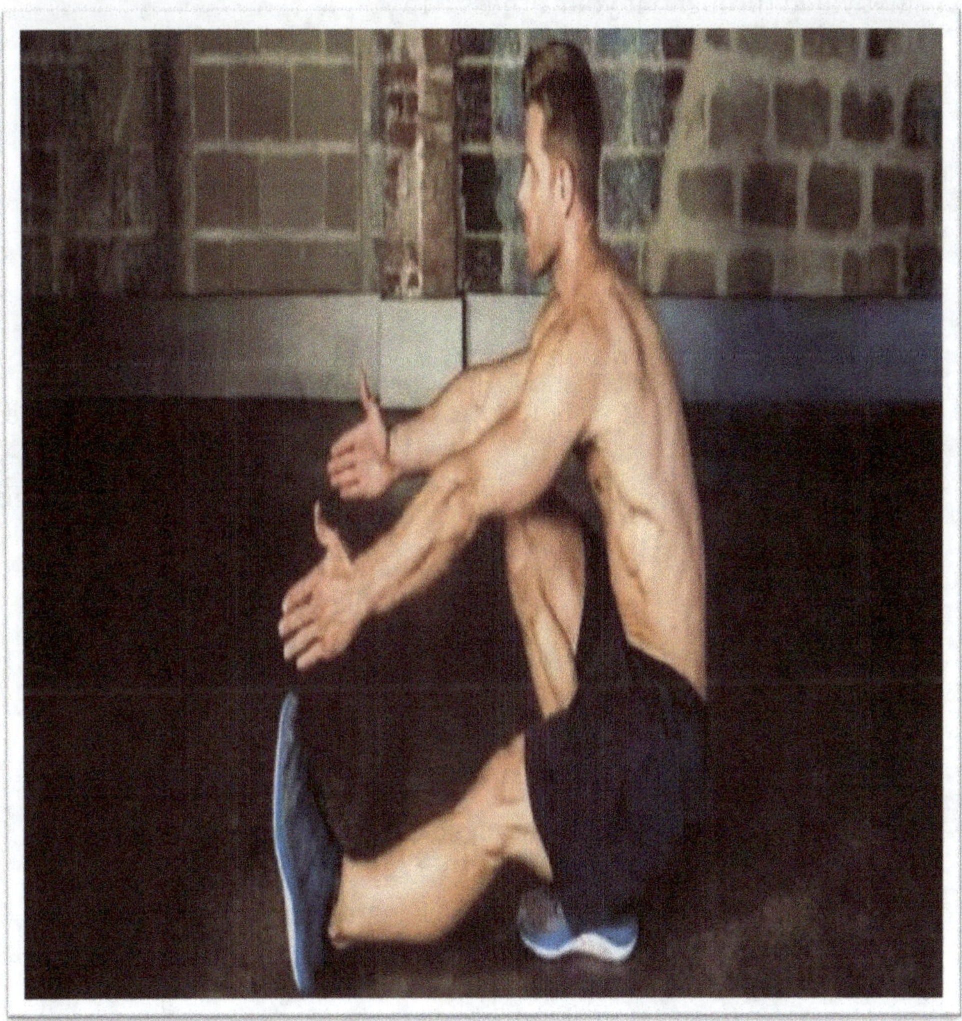

Embarking on a fitness trip is an instigative bid, but maintaining provocation and shadowing progress can be challenging over time. Whether you are aiming to lose weight, make muscle, or ameliorate your overall health, enforcing effective strategies for covering your progress and staying motivated is essential for long-term success.

Then is a comprehensive companion to tracking progress and staying motivated throughout your fitness trip

Set SMART pretensions

Specific easily define your pretensions, making them specific and measurable. For illustration, rather than saying "I want to lose weight" specify how important weight you aim to lose and in what timeframe.

Measurable Use ideal criteria to track your progress, similar as pounds lost, elevation gained, or advancements in strength or abidance.

Attainable Set pretensions that are realistic and attainable grounded on your current fitness position, life, and coffers.

Applicable insure your pretensions align with your values and precedence's, keeping them applicable and meaningful to you.

Time- bound Establish deadlines or target dates for achieving your pretensions, furnishing a sense of urgency and responsibility.

Keep a Workout Journal

Track your exercises, including the exercises performed, sets, reps, weights, and any notes or compliances.

Record other applicable data similar as your body weight, measures, and how you feel before, during, and after exercise sessions.

Review your journal regularly to identify patterns, track progress over time, and celebrate achievements.

Fitness Apps and Wearable Technology

Take advantage of fitness apps and wearable bias to track your exertion situations, cover heart rate, calories burned, and other applicable criteria.

Set monuments, pretensions, and challenges within these apps to keep you responsible and motivated.

Numerous apps offer social features that allow you to connect with musketeers, share progress, and contend in challenges, fostering a sense of community and support.

Find Responsibility mates

Partner up with musketeers, family members, or associates who partake in analogous fitness pretensions and interests.

Schedule regular check- sways, exercises, or challenges together to hold each other responsible and give collective support and stimulant.

Join online communities, forums, or social media groups concentrated on fitness and heartiness to connect with suchlike- inclined individualities and share gests.

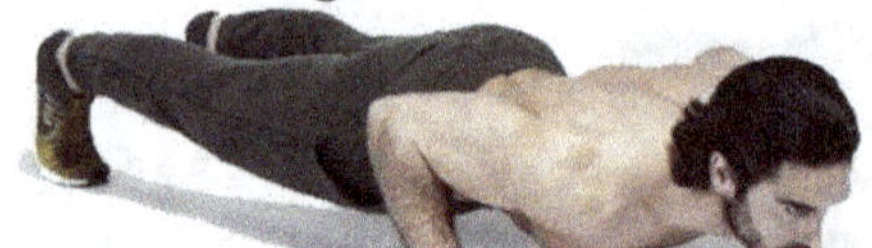

Price Yourself for mileposts

Set up a system of prices for achieving mileposts along your fitness trip, whether it's reaching a certain weight, completing a specific number of exercises, or hitting a particular stylish in performance.

Prices can be anything that motivates you, similar as treating yourself to a massage, buying new drill gear, or enjoying a cheat mess.

Stay Inspired and Educated

Seek alleviation from part models, success stories, and fitness influencers who have achieved analogous pretensions.

Educate yourself about fitness, nutrition, and heartiness through books, podcasts, papers, and estimable online coffers.

Try new drill routines exercises and conditioning, to keep your exercises fresh and instigative.

Embrace Inflexibility and Rigidity

Be flexible and adaptable in your approach to fitness, feting that progress may not always follow a direct path.

Acclimating your pretension routines and prospects as demanded, grounded on changes in circumstances, precedencies, or preferences.

Practice Self- Compassion and tolerance

Be kind to yourself and admit that lapses and obstacles are a natural part of the trip.

Practice tone- compassion and adaptability, fastening on progress rather than perfection.

Celebrate small palms along the way and remind yourself of how far you've come.

Enforcing these strategies for tracking progress and staying motivated, you will empower yourself to navigate the ups and campo of your fitness trip with confidence, adaptability, and determination. Flash back that success isn't defined by a destination but by the trip itself, and each step you take brings you near to getting the stylish interpretation of yourself.

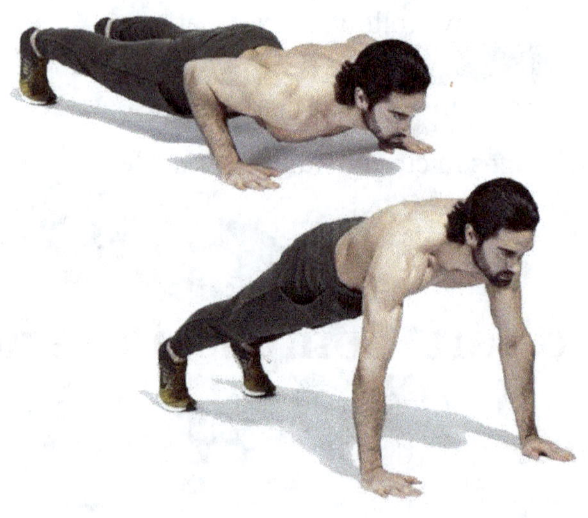

8

Nutrition Tips for Supporting Your Fitness Journey

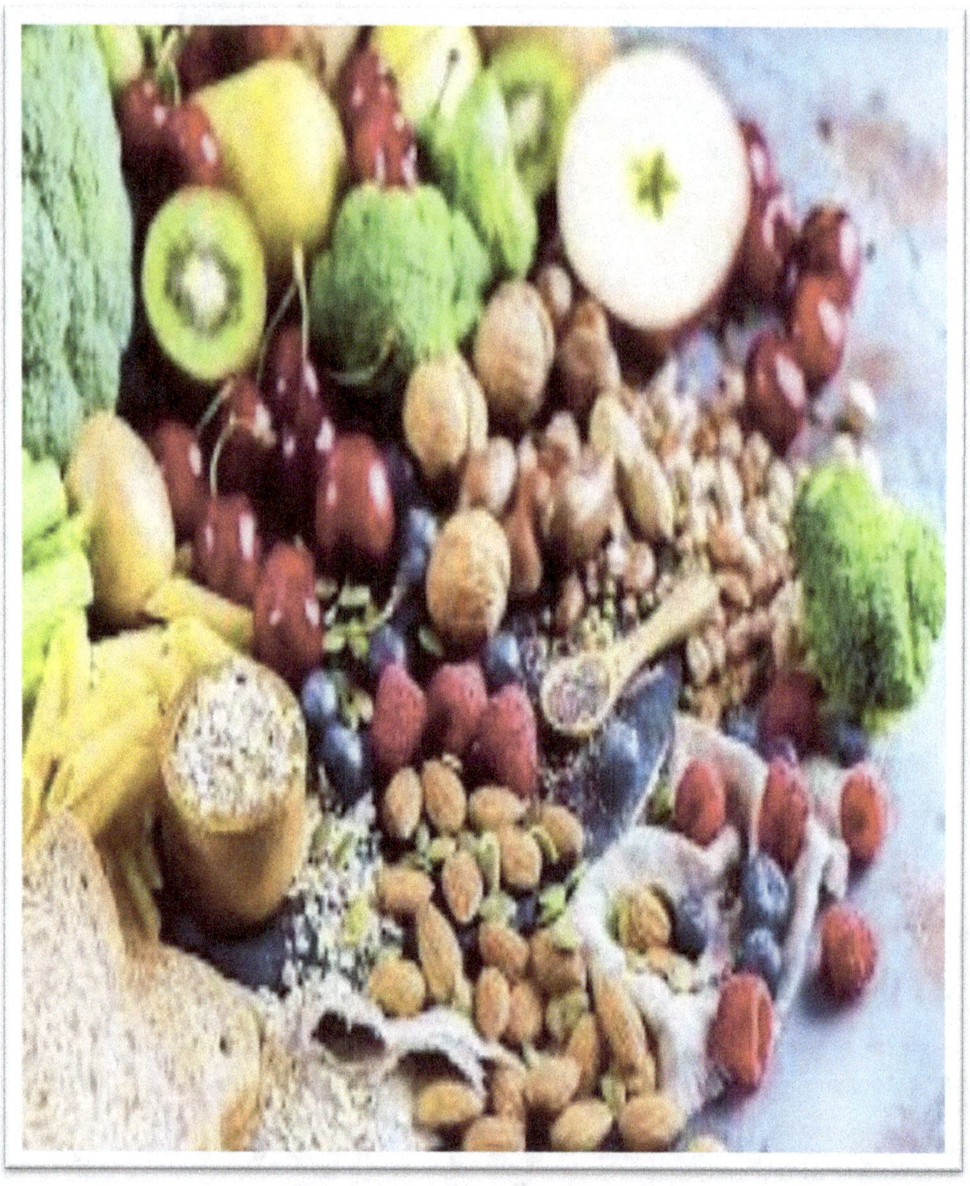

P roper nutrition plays a fundamental role in fueling your body for exercise, supporting recovery, and maximizing performance. Whether your fitness goals include losing weight, building muscle, or improving overall health and well-being, adopting a balanced and nutrient-rich diet is essential. Here are some nutrition tips to support your fitness journey

Prioritize Whole, Nutrient-Dense Foods

Base your meals and snacks around whole, minimally processed foods such as fruits, vegetables, lean proteins, whole grains, nuts, seeds, and legumes.

These foods provide essential vitamins, minerals, antioxidants, fiber, and macronutrients (carbohydrates, proteins, and fats) necessary for optimal health and performance.

Balance Macronutrients

Aim to include a balance of carbohydrates, proteins, and healthy fats in each meal to provide sustained energy, support muscle repair and growth, and regulate metabolism.

Choose complex carbohydrates (e.g., whole grains, fruits and vegetables) for sustained energy, lean proteins (e.g., chicken, fish, tofu, beans) for muscle repair and satiety, and healthy fats (e.g., avocado, nuts and olive oil) for heart health and hormone regulation.

Fuel Your Workouts

Eat a balanced meal or snack containing carbohydrates and protein 1-3 hours before exercise to fuel your workouts and optimize performance.

Choose easily digestible options such as a banana with almond butter, Greek yogurt with berries, or a turkey and avocado sandwich on whole grain bread.

Hydrate Properly

Stay adequately hydrated before, during, and after exercise to maintain optimal performance, prevent dehydration, and support recovery.

Drink water throughout the day and consider consuming electrolyte-rich beverages or snacks during prolonged or intense workouts to replace lost fluids and minerals.

Timing Your Meals and Snacks

Eat balanced meals and snacks every 3-4 hours to keep energy levels steady and prevent dips in blood sugar.

Refuel with a combination of carbohydrates and protein within 30-60 minutes post-workout to replenish glycogen stores, repair muscle tissue, and promote recovery.

Listen to Your Body

Pay attention to hunger and satiety cues, eating when you're hungry and stopping when you're satisfied.

Practice mindful eating, savoring each bite, and tuning in to how different foods make you feel physically and emotionally.

Plan and Prepare

Plan your meals and snacks ahead of time, making sure to include a variety of nutrient-rich foods to meet your dietary needs and preferences.

Batch cook and meal prep ingredients in advance to streamline mealtime and ensure you have healthy options readily available, especially during busy periods.

Avoid Restrictive Diets

Avoid fad diets or overly restrictive eating patterns that may compromise your nutritional intake, lead to nutrient deficiencies, and negatively impact your energy levels and performance.

Instead, focus on creating a sustainable and balanced approach to eating that nourishes your body and supports your long-term health and fitness goals.

Seek Professional Guidance

Consider consulting with a registered dietitian or nutritionist who specializes in sports nutrition to receive personalized guidance and recommendations tailored to your individual needs, goals, and dietary preferences.

Incorporate these nutrition tips into your lifestyle, you'll provide your body with the essential nutrients it needs to thrive, support your fitness goals, and enhance your overall health and well-being.

Remember that nutrition is a key component of your fitness journey, and making mindful choices around food can have a significant impact on your success and longevity in reaching your goals.

9

Incorporating Rest and Recovery

Essential Components of a Balanced Fitness Routine

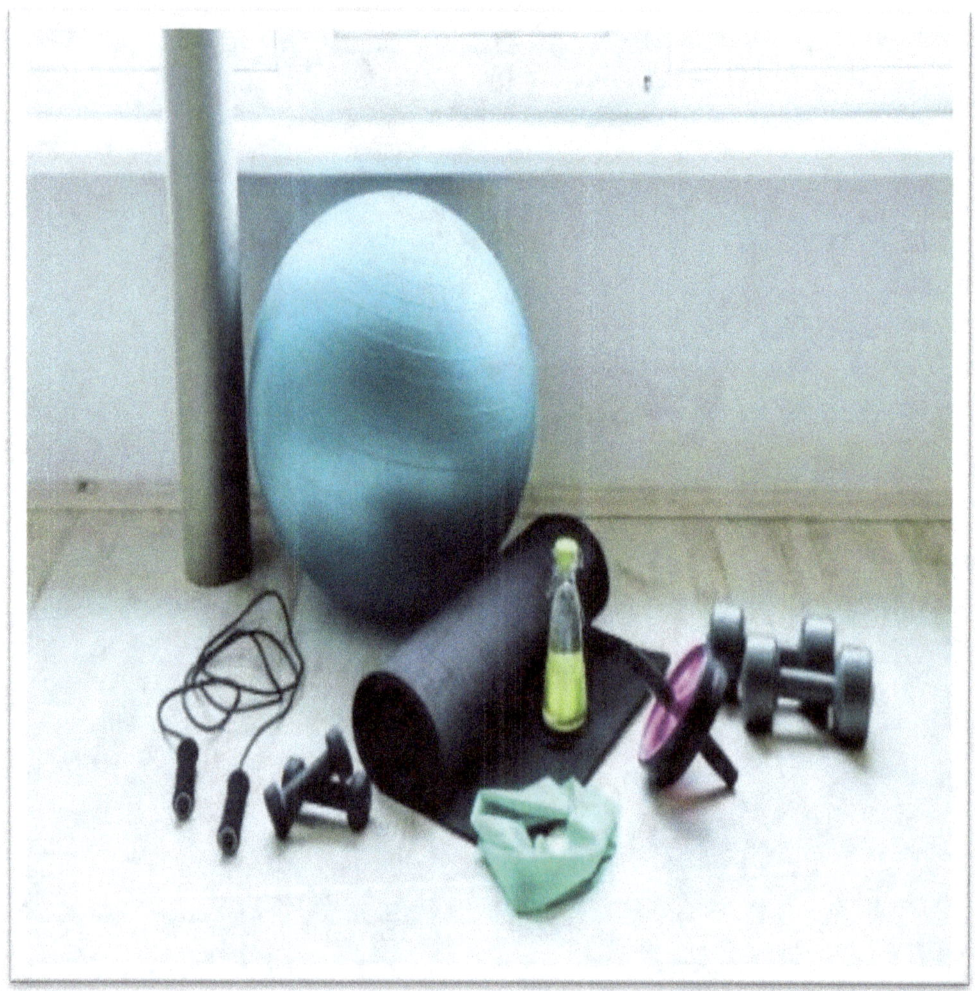

In the pursuit of fitness pretensions, numerous individualities concentrate primarily on exercise intensity and frequencies while overlooking the critical significance of rest and recovery. Still, acceptable rest and recovery are essential for optimizing performance, precluding injury, and promoting overall well- being.

Then is a comprehensive companion to incorporating rest and recovery into your fitness routine.

Understand the significance of Rest Days

Rest days are essential for allowing your body to recover from the physical stress of exercise, form muscle towel, and replenish energy stores.

Plan regular rest days into your drill schedule, aiming for at least one or two days of complete rest per week.

Hear to your body and acclimate your rest days grounded on your energy situations, muscle soreness, and overall recovery requirements.

Practice Active Recovery

On rest days, engage in low- intensity conditioning similar as walking, gentle yoga, swimming, or cycling to promote blood inflow, reduce muscle stiffness, and enhance recovery.

Active recovery helps flush out metabolic waste products from your muscles, accelerates the mending process, and aids in reducing post-exercise soreness.

Get Acceptable Sleep

Prioritize quality sleep as an integral part of your recovery routine, aiming for 7- 9 hours of continued sleep per night

Sleep is pivotal for muscle form, hormone regulation, cognitive function, and overall physical and internal well- being.

Produce a sleep-friendly terrain by minimizing exposure to defenses, establishing a harmonious sleep schedule, and rehearsing relaxation ways before bedtime.

Hear to Your Body

Pay attention to signs of overtraining, including patient fatigue, dropped performance, increased vulnerability to illness, and mood disturbances.

If you witness symptoms of overtraining, gauge back your exercises, increase rest days, and prioritize recovery conditioning similar as froth rolling, stretching, and massage.

Nutrition for Recovery

Support your body's recovery process by consuming nutrient-rich foods that give essential vitamins, minerals, and macronutrients.

Include high- quality protein sources, complex carbohydrates, healthy fats, and plenitude of fruits and vegetables in your post-workout refection and snacks to replenish glycogen stores, form muscle towel, and promote recovery.

Hydration

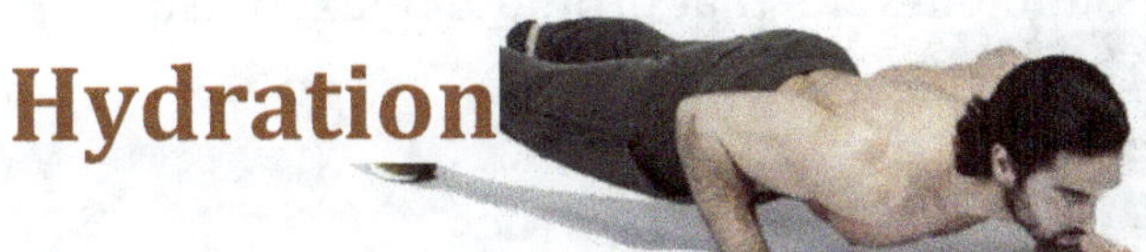

Stay adequately doused before, during, and after exercise to support optimal performance and recovery

Water is essential for maintaining proper hydration, regulating body temperature, and easing the transport of nutrients and oxygen to your muscles.

Incorporate Recovery ways

Use colorful recovery ways similar as froth rolling, massage, discrepancy cataracts, and stretching to palliate muscle pressure, ameliorate inflexibility, and enhance recovery.

Try different recovery modalities to find what works best for your body and preferences.

Mental and Emotional Recovery

Fete the significance of internal and emotional recovery in your overall well- being.

Practice stress operation ways similar as awareness, contemplation, deep breathing exercises, and pursuits that promote relaxation and enjoyment.

Schedule Deload Weeks

Periodically incorporate deload weeks into your training schedule, during which you reduce training volume and intensity to allow for extended recovery and help collapse.

Deload weeks can help overtraining, promote physical and internal revivification, and insure long- term progress and sustainability in your fitness trip.

Prioritizing rest and recovery as integral factors of your fitness routine, you will optimize your performance, reduce the threat of injury, and support your overall health and well- being.

Flash back that progress isn't just about pushing harder but also about allowing your-self the time and space to rest, recover, and rejuvenate for uninterrupted success and life in your fitness trip.

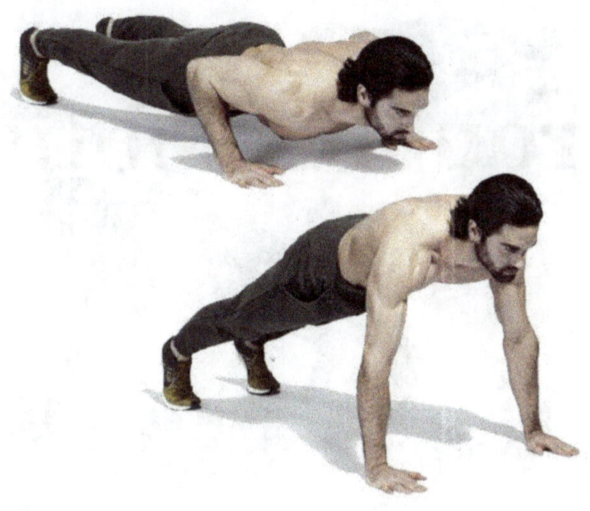

10

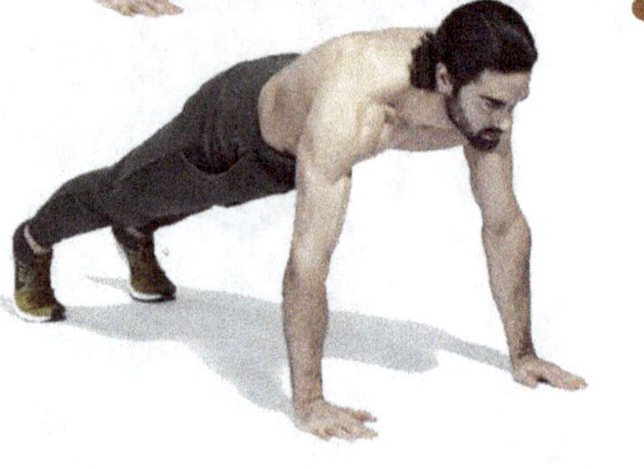

Troubleshooting

Common Challenges in Your Fitness Journey

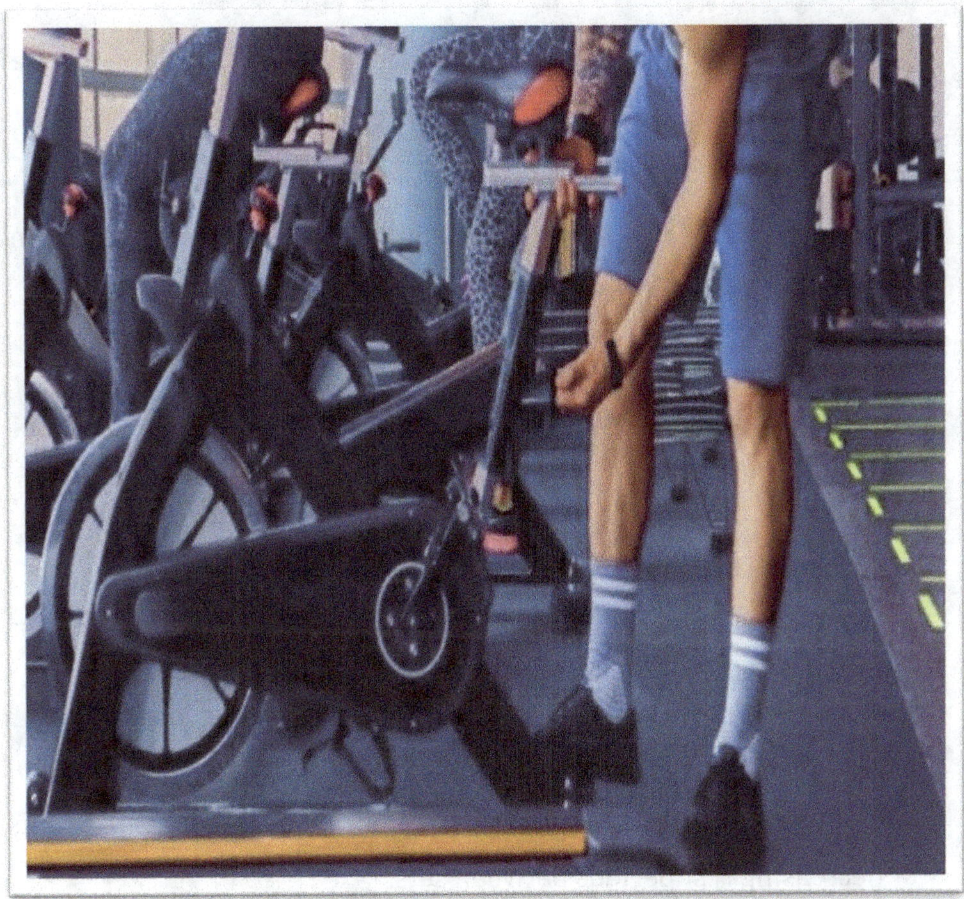

Embarking on a fitness journey is an exciting endeavor filled with opportunities for growth and transformation. However, it's not uncommon to encounter challenges along the way that can hinder progress and dampen motivation.

identifying and addressing these common obstacles proactively, you can overcome setbacks and stay on track towards achieving your goals. Here's a comprehensive guide to troubleshooting common challenges in your fitness journey.

Overcoming Plateaus

Plateaus occur when your progress stalls despite consistent effort and adherence to your fitness regimen.

To overcome plateaus, consider implementing changes to your workout routine, such as increasing the intensity, duration, or frequency of your workouts.

Incorporate variety into your workouts by trying new exercises, workout modalities, or training techniques to shock your body out of its comfort zone.

Focus on progressive overload, gradually increasing the challenge to your muscles by lifting heavier weights, performing more repetitions, or decreasing rest periods between sets.

Dealing with Soreness

Delayed onset muscle soreness (DOMS) is common, especially when starting a new workout program or increasing the intensity of your workouts.

To alleviate soreness, prioritize adequate warm-up and cool-down routines, engage in gentle stretching and foam rolling, and consider taking rest days or engaging in active recovery activities.

Listen to your body and avoid pushing through excessive pain, as this can lead to further injury and delay recovery.

Adjusting Your Routine for Injury or Illness

Injuries and illnesses can disrupt your fitness routine and require modifications to prevent further damage and promote healing.

If you're injured or ill, prioritize rest and recovery, and avoid activities that exacerbate your condition.

Consult with a healthcare professional or physical therapist for guidance on appropriate exercises and rehabilitation protocols to safely return to activity.

Focus on maintaining a positive mindset and staying patient throughout the recovery process, understanding that setbacks are temporary and part of the journey.

Managing Time Constraints

Balancing work, family obligations, and other commitments can make it challenging to find time for exercise.

Prioritize scheduling workouts as you would any other important appointment, and consider early morning or evening workouts to accommodate your schedule.

Incorporate short, high-intensity workouts or interval training sessions that provide maximum benefit in minimal time.

Look for opportunities to integrate physical activity into your daily routine, such as taking the stairs instead of the elevator or going for a walk during your lunch break.

Overcoming Mental Barriers

Mental barriers such as self-doubt fear of failure, or lack of motivation can impede progress and hinder your ability to reach your fitness goals.

Practice positive self-talk and cultivate a growth mindset, focusing on progress rather than perfection.

Set realistic and achievable goals, breaking them down into smaller, manageable steps to build confidence and momentum.

Surround yourself with a supportive community of like-minded individuals who inspire and motivate you to stay committed to your fitness journey.

Finding Balance and Sustainability

Striking a balance between fitness goals and other aspects of life, such as work, relationships, and hobbies, is essential for long-term sustainability.

Prioritize self-care and listen to your body's signals, allowing for adequate rest, recovery, and enjoyment outside of exercise.

Practice flexibility in your approach to fitness, adjusting your routine as needed to accommodate changing circumstances and priorities.

Focus on building healthy habits that are sustainable over the long term, rather than pursuing short-term results at the expense of your overall well-being.

Recognizing and addressing these common challenges in your fitness journey, you'll develop resilience, perseverance, and a greater sense of self-awareness that will propel you towards success and fulfillment in reaching your goals. Remember that setbacks are temporary and opportunities for growth and by staying committed to your journey, you'll emerge stronger, healthier, and more empowered than ever before.

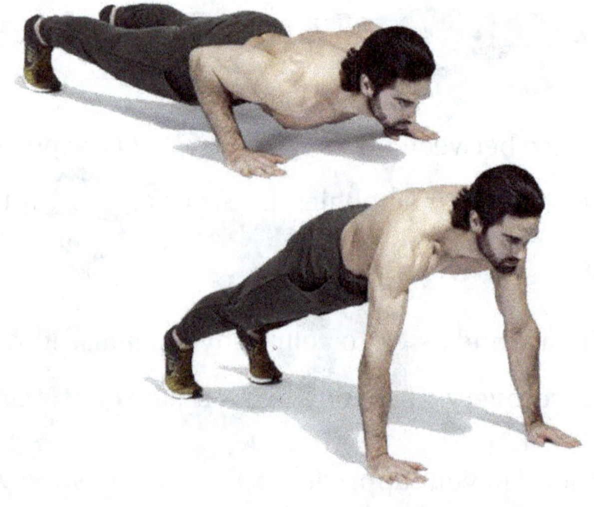

11

Seeking Further Resources

Expanding Your Knowledge and Support Network

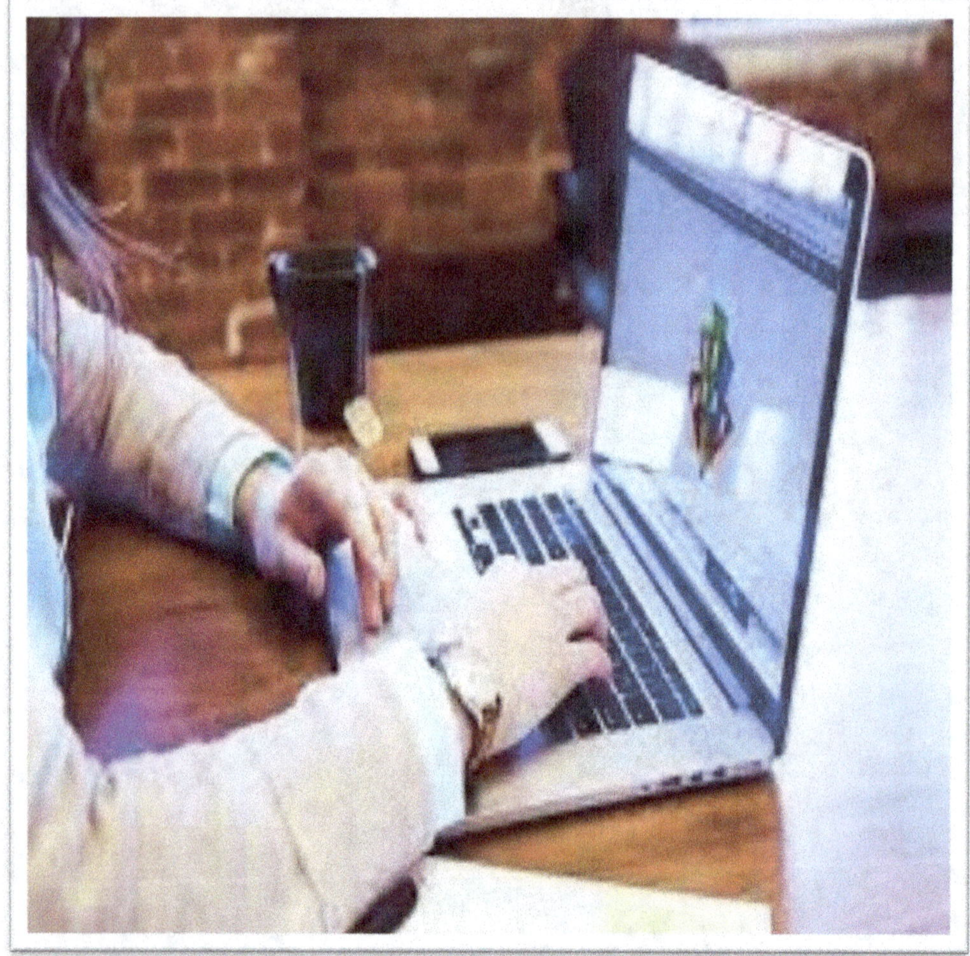

Embarking on a fitness journey can be both exciting and overwhelming, especially with the abundance of information and resources available. Whether you're looking to deepen your understanding of exercise science, explore new workout routines, or connect with like-minded individuals, seeking further resources can enhance your journey and empower you to reach your fitness goals. Here's a comprehensive guide to expanding your knowledge and support network.

Online Resources

Explore reputable websites, blogs, and forums dedicated to fitness, nutrition, and wellness. Websites such as Bodybuilding.com, ACE Fitness, and the American Council on Exercise (ACE) offer a wealth of articles, workout plans, and expert advice.

Follow fitness influencers, trainers, and experts on social media platforms such as Instagram, YouTube, and TikTok for workout tips, motivation, and inspiration.

Join online communities and forums such as Reddit's r/fitness or fitness-related Facebook groups to connect with individuals who share similar goals and interests.

Books and Publications

Dive deeper into specific topics related to fitness, nutrition, and exercise science by reading books written by experts in the field. Look for titles recommended by reputable sources or authors with recognized credentials.

Consider subscribing to fitness magazines such as Men's Health, Women's Health, or Muscle & Fitness for regular updates on the latest trends, workouts, and nutrition tips.

Podcasts and Audio Resources

Listen to podcasts focused on fitness, health, and wellness during your workouts, commute, or downtime. Podcasts such as The Model Health Show, The Strength Running Podcast, and The Mind Pump Podcast cover a wide range of topics related to fitness and lifestyle optimization.

Audible and other audiobook platforms offer a vast selection of audiobooks on fitness, nutrition, and personal development, allowing you to absorb valuable information while on the go.

Continuing Education and Certifications

Consider pursuing formal education or certifications in fitness-related fields if you're passionate about deepening your knowledge and potentially turning your interest into a career. Organizations such as ACE, NASM, and ISSA offer accredited certification programs for personal trainers, fitness instructors, and health coaches.

Attend workshops, seminars, and conferences led by industry experts to stay updated on the latest research, trends, and best practices in fitness and wellness.

Professional Guidance and Coaching

Invest in personalized guidance and support from certified fitness professionals, nutritionists, or health coaches who can tailor recommendations to your individual needs and goals.

Work with a personal trainer or coach to design a customized workout program, receive accountability and motivation, and ensure proper form and technique during exercise sessions.

Consider seeking guidance from a registered dietitian or nutritionist for personalized nutrition counseling, meal planning, and dietary recommendations to support your fitness goals.

Local Resources and Facilities

Explore local gyms, fitness studios, and community centers in your area that offer group fitness classes, personal training services, and wellness programs.

Participate in group fitness classes such as yoga, Pilates, spinning, or HIIT workouts to add variety to your routine and connect with others in your community who share similar interests.

Wellness Apps and Technology

Utilize fitness apps, trackers, and wearable devices to monitor your progress, track workouts, and stay motivated. Popular apps such as MyFitnessPal, Strava, and Fitbit offer features for logging workouts, tracking nutrition, and setting goals.

Experiment with virtual fitness platforms and streaming services that offer on-demand workout classes, live coaching sessions, and personalized training programs, allowing you to exercise from the comfort of your own home.

Seeking further resources and expanding your knowledge and support network, you'll gain valuable insights, tools, and connections that will enrich your fitness journey and empower you to achieve your goals with confidence and success. Remember to approach information with a critical mindset, prioritize reputable sources, and experiment with different strategies to find what works best for you.

Conclusion

Empowering Your Fitness Journey

Embarking on a fitness trip is a transformative bid that extends far beyond physical changes — it's a trip of tone- discovery, adaptability, and particular growth.

Throughout this companion, we have explored essential aspects of fitness, from exercise basics to nutrition tips, rest and recovery strategies, and troubleshooting common challenges.

By equipping yourself with knowledge, tools, and strategies, you've taken the first way towards realizing your fitness pretensions and unleashing your full eventuality.

As you navigate your fitness trip, flash back that progress isn't always direct, and lapses are a natural part of the process. Embrace challenges as openings for growth, and approach your trip with tolerance, perseverance, and a positive mindset.

Celebrate small palms along the way, and admit the strength and adaptability you've formerly demonstrated in committing to your health and well- being.

Likewise, fete the significance of tone- care and balance in maintaining a sustainable fitness routine.

Hear to your body's signals, prioritize rest and recovery, and foster a holistic approach to health that encompasses physical, internal, and emotional well- being.

Compass yourself with a probative community of like- inclined individualities who inspire and motivate you to stay married to your pretensions.

As you continue on your fitness trip, know that you aren't alone. There are innumerous coffers available to support and guide you along the way, from fitness apps and online communities to fitness professionals, Nutritionist and healthcare providers do not vacillate to seek farther coffers and support as demanded, and flash back that asking for help is a sign of strength, not weakness.

Above all, trust in yourself and your capability to overcome obstacles, achieve your pretensions, and live a life of vitality and purpose. Your fitness trip is a reflection of your inner strength, determination, and commitment to getting the stylish interpretation of your-self.

Embrace the trip, embrace the challenges, and embrace the inconceivable eventuality that lies within you.

Then it is to your uninterrupted success of growth and commission on your fitness trip.

May you embrace every step, every challenge, and every triumph with courage, adaptability, and unwavering determination? You've got this!

* 9 7 9 8 3 2 3 2 4 5 6 8 0 *